Nursing Student Weekly Planner
with Pharmacology Study Notes
January 2019-May 2020

This planner is a product of Andrea's Notes

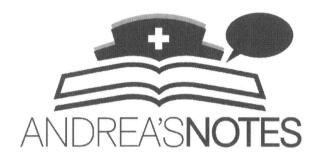

andreasnotes.com

ISBN-13: 978-1719241328
ISBN-10: 1719241325

2019

January

Su	Mo	Tu	We	Th	Fr	Sa
	1	2	3	4	5	
6	7	8	9	10	11	12
13	14	15	16	17	18	19
20	21	22	23	24	25	26
27	28	29	30	31		

February

Su	Mo	Tu	We	Th	Fr	Sa
					1	2
3	4	5	6	7	8	9
10	11	12	13	14	15	16
17	18	19	20	21	22	23
24	25	26	27	28		

March

Su	Mo	Tu	We	Th	Fr	Sa
					1	2
3	4	5	6	7	8	9
10	11	12	13	14	15	16
17	18	19	20	21	22	23
24	25	26	27	28	29	30
31						

April

Su	Mo	Tu	We	Th	Fr	Sa
	1	2	3	4	5	6
7	8	9	10	11	12	13
14	15	16	17	18	19	20
21	22	23	24	25	26	27
28	29	30				

May

Su	Mo	Tu	We	Th	Fr	Sa
			1	2	3	4
5	6	7	8	9	10	11
12	13	14	15	16	17	18
19	20	21	22	23	24	25
26	27	28	29	30	31	

June

Su	Mo	Tu	We	Th	Fr	Sa
						1
2	3	4	5	6	7	8
9	10	11	12	13	14	15
16	17	18	19	20	21	22
23	24	25	26	27	28	29
30						

July

Su	Mo	Tu	We	Th	Fr	Sa
	1	2	3	4	5	6
7	8	9	10	11	12	13
14	15	16	17	18	19	20
21	22	23	24	25	26	27
28	29	30	31			

August

Su	Mo	Tu	We	Th	Fr	Sa
				1	2	3
4	5	6	7	8	9	10
11	12	13	14	15	16	17
18	19	20	21	22	23	24
25	26	27	28	29	30	31

September

Su	Mo	Tu	We	Th	Fr	Sa
1	2	3	4	5	6	7
8	9	10	11	12	13	14
15	16	17	18	19	20	21
22	23	24	25	26	27	28
29	30					

October

Su	Mo	Tu	We	Th	Fr	Sa
		1	2	3	4	5
6	7	8	9	10	11	12
13	14	15	16	17	18	19
20	21	22	23	24	25	26
27	28	29	30	31		

November

Su	Mo	Tu	We	Th	Fr	Sa
					1	2
3	4	5	6	7	8	9
10	11	12	13	14	15	16
17	18	19	20	21	22	23
24	25	26	27	28	29	30

December

Su	Mo	Tu	We	Th	Fr	Sa
1	2	3	4	5	6	7
8	9	10	11	12	13	14
15	16	17	18	19	20	21
22	23	24	25	26	27	28
29	30	31				

2020

January

Su	Mo	Tu	We	Th	Fr	Sa
			1	2	3	4
5	6	7	8	9	10	11
12	13	14	15	16	17	18
19	20	21	22	23	24	25
26	27	28	29	30	31	

February

Su	Mo	Tu	We	Th	Fr	Sa
						1
2	3	4	5	6	7	8
9	10	11	12	13	14	15
16	17	18	19	20	21	22
23	24	25	26	27	28	29

March

Su	Mo	Tu	We	Th	Fr	Sa
1	2	3	4	5	6	7
8	9	10	11	12	13	14
15	16	17	18	19	20	21
22	23	24	25	26	27	28
29	30	31				

April

Su	Mo	Tu	We	Th	Fr	Sa
			1	2	3	4
5	6	7	8	9	10	11
12	13	14	15	16	17	18
19	20	21	22	23	24	25
26	27	28	29	30		

May

Su	Mo	Tu	We	Th	Fr	Sa
					1	2
3	4	5	6	7	8	9
10	11	12	13	14	15	16
17	18	19	20	21	22	23
24	25	26	27	28	29	30
31						

June

Su	Mo	Tu	We	Th	Fr	Sa
	1	2	3	4	5	6
7	8	9	10	11	12	13
14	15	16	17	18	19	20
21	22	23	24	25	26	27
28	29	30				

July

Su	Mo	Tu	We	Th	Fr	Sa
			1	2	3	4
5	6	7	8	9	10	11
12	13	14	15	16	17	18
19	20	21	22	23	24	25
26	27	28	29	30	31	

August

Su	Mo	Tu	We	Th	Fr	Sa
						1
2	3	4	5	6	7	8
9	10	11	12	13	14	15
16	17	18	19	20	21	22
23	24	25	26	27	28	29
30	31					

September

Su	Mo	Tu	We	Th	Fr	Sa
		1	2	3	4	5
6	7	8	9	10	11	12
13	14	15	16	17	18	19
20	21	22	23	24	25	26
27	28	29	30			

October

Su	Mo	Tu	We	Th	Fr	Sa
				1	2	3
4	5	6	7	8	9	10
11	12	13	14	15	16	17
18	19	20	21	22	23	24
25	26	27	28	29	30	31

November

Su	Mo	Tu	We	Th	Fr	Sa
1	2	3	4	5	6	7
8	9	10	11	12	13	14
15	16	17	18	19	20	21
22	23	24	25	26	27	28
29	30					

December

Su	Mo	Tu	We	Th	Fr	Sa
		1	2	3	4	5
6	7	8	9	10	11	12
13	14	15	16	17	18	19
20	21	22	23	24	25	26
27	28	29	30	31		

Pharmacology Study Notes

Topic	Month
Angiotensin Converting Enzyme (ACE) Inhibitors	Jan. 2019
Antianxiety Agents	Jan.
Anticoagulants	Jan/Feb
Anticonvulsants	Feb
Antidepressants – SSRIs	Feb/March
Antidepressants – SNRIs	March/April
Antidiabetic – Insulins	May
Antidiabetic Oral Medications	June
Antihistamines	June/July
Anti-Infectives – Cephalosporin	July
Anti-Infectives - Fluoroquinolone	July
Anti-Infectives – Macrolide	August
Anti-Infectives – Penicillin	August
Anti-Infectives – Sulfonamide	August
Anti-Infectives – Tetracycline	September
Antipsychotics	Sept/Oct
Antiulcer Agents	October
Asthma Medications	Oct/Nov
Beta Blockers	Nov/Dec
Calcium Channel Blockers (CCBs)	Dec/Jan
Corticosteroid	January 2020
Diuretics	Feb
Lipid-Lowering Agents	Feb/March
Non-Steroidal Anti-Inflammatory Drugs (NSAIDS)	March
Sedatives / Hypnotics	April
Skeletal Muscle Relaxants	April/May

January

Sunday	Monday	Tuesday	Wednesday
		1 New Year's Day	2
6	7	8	9
13	14	15	16
20	21 M L King Day	22	23
27	28	29	30

NCLEX Review Question

A patient who has just been prescribed lisinopril (Prinvil) for heart failure asks you how the drug will work. What is your best response?

A. It will slow your heart rate
B. It will cause your arteries to constrict
C. It will decrease the fluid and sodium in your blood
D. It will increase the strength of your heart contractions

Correct Answer: C.

2019

Thursday	Friday	Saturday	Notes
3	4	5	
10	11	12	
17	18	19	
24	25	26	
31			

NCLEX Review Question

The nurse is caring for a patient who is prescribed enalapril (Vasotec) 5mg daily. For which life-threatening adverse effect does the nurse assess the patient?

A. Angioedema
B. Endocarditis
C. Hepatitis
D. Encephalitis

Correct Answer: A.

January
2019

Monday	

Tuesday 1	

Wednesday 2	

Angiotensin Converting Enzyme (ACE) Inhibitors

Most commonly prescribed:

☞ benazepril (Lotensin)

☞ enalapril (Vasotec)

☞ lisinopril (Prinvil, Zestril)

January
2019

Thursday **3**	
Friday **4**	
Sat **5**	
Sun **6**	

Notes

January
2019

Monday 7	
Tuesday 8	
Wednesday 9	

Angiotensin Converting Enzyme (ACE) Inhibitors

Uses:

☞ Treat mild to moderate hypertension, heart failure, and prevent stroke

Nursing Considerations:

☞ Advise patients to change positions (lying, sitting, standing) slowly to avoid orthostatic hypotension

☞ Medications can cause a permanent dry cough

January
2019

Thursday **10**	
Friday **11**	
Sat **12**	
Sun **13**	

Notes

January
2019

Monday **14**	
Tuesday **15**	
Wednesday **16**	

Antianxiety Agents

Most commonly prescribed:

- alprazolam (Xanax)
- diazepam (Valium)
- lorazepam (Ativan)
- paroxetine (Paxil)
- venlafaxine (Effexor)

January
2019

Thursday **17**	
Friday **18**	
Sat **19**	
Sun **20**	

Notes

January
2019

Monday 21	

Tuesday 22	

Wednesday 23	

Antianxiety Agents

Uses:

🎗 Treat generalized anxiety disorder and panic disorder

🎗 Manage anxiety related to depression

Nursing Considerations:

🎗 Benzodiazepines such as diazepam may be used to treat alcohol withdrawal and seizures – may also be habit forming

🎗 Patients should NOT stop medication abruptly – may cause seizures

🎗 Patients should avoid CNS depressants such as alcohol

January
2019

Thursday 24	
Friday 25	
Sat 26	
Sun 27	

Notes

January
2019

Monday **28**	
Tuesday **29**	
Wednesday **30**	

Anticoagulants

Most commonly prescribed:

dabigatran (Pradaxa)

warfarin (Coumadin)

January/February
2019

Thursday 31	
Friday **1**	
Sat **2**	
Sun **3**	

Notes

February

Sunday	Monday	Tuesday	Wednesday
3	4	5	6
10	11	12	13
17	18 Presidents' Day	19 1st care plan due: before 6:29 am	20
24	25	26	27

NCLEX Review Question

The nurse caring for a patient with a warfarin (Coumadin) overdose anticipates the prescriber to order which medication for the patient?

- A. Protamine sulfate
- B. Potassium
- C. Vitamin K
- D. Vitamin C

Correct Answer: C.

2019

Thursday	Friday	Saturday	Notes
	1	2	
7	8	9	
14 exam #2 Valentine's Day	15	16	
21	22	23	
28 exam #3 meet w/ Porter 0920			

NCLEX Review Question

A nurse is caring for a patient with a new order for continuous IV heparin therapy. Which action should the nurse take first?

- A. Make a sign stating, "No IM or SQ injections"
- B. Obtain patient's accurate baseline weight
- C. Draw INR blood test and send to lab stat
- D. Instruct patient to remain on bedrest

Correct Answer: B.

February
2019

Monday **4**	
Tuesday **5**	
Wednesday **6**	

Anticoagulants

Uses:

May treat or prevent blood clots from forming or getting bigger while your body slowly reabsorbs the clot. Patients with a history of stroke, myocardial infarction (heart attack), valvular disease, coronary artery disease, heart failure, arrhythmia, atrial fibrillation (a-fib), deep vein thrombosis (DVT) and pulmonary embolism are at increased risk for blood clots.

February
2019

Thursday **7**	
Friday **8**	
Sat **9**	
Sun **10**	

Notes

February
2019

Monday **11**	
Tuesday **12**	
Wednesday **13**	

Anticoagulants

Nursing Considerations:

Increased risk for bleeding, so monitor for bleeding gums, epistaxis (nosebleed), black or tarry stools

Advise patient to wear a medical alert tag

Inform patient that foods rich in vitamin K such as green leafy veggies can reduce the effectiveness of the medication

February
2019

Thursday **14**	
Friday **15**	
Sat **16**	
Sun **17**	

Notes

February
2019

Monday 18	No school
Tuesday 19	first care plan due @ clinical
Wednesday 20	

Anticoagulants

Nursing Considerations:
Certain herbal remedies may change medication effect – Ginseng & St. John's Wort may decrease PT/INR, while Ginkgo biloba, garlic, chamomile and licorice may increase PT/INR lab values.

February
2019

Thursday 21	
Friday 22	
Sat 23	
Sun 24	

Notes

February
2019

Monday 25	
Monday **25**	
Tuesday **26**	- Official Assessment - Clinical
Wednesday **27**	

Anticonvulsants

Most commonly prescribed:

🫀 clonazepam (Klonopin)

🫀 diazepam (Valium)

🫀 gabapentin (Neurontin)

🫀 pregabalin (Lyrica)

February/March
2019

Thursday 28	exam#3
	meet w/ Porter 0920-0940
Friday 1	
Sat 2	
Sun 3	

Notes

March

Sunday	Monday	Tuesday	Wednesday
3	4	5	6
10	11	12	13
17	18	19	20
24	25	26	27
31			

NCLEX Review Question

A nurse caring for a patient who is prescribed gabapentin (Neurontin) for seizures and aluminum hydroxide (Amphojel) for indigestion, would instruct the patient to:

A. Take the gabapentin 1 hour after the aluminum hydroxide.
B. Take the gabapentin 2 hours after the aluminum hydroxide.
C. Take these two drugs together for the best action of both drugs
D . Ask the provider for a different antacid to avoid a drug interaction

Correct Answer: B.

2019

Thursday	Friday	Saturday	Notes
	1	2	
7	8	9	
14	15	16	
21	22	23	
28	29	30	

NCLEX Review Question

A nursing caring for a patient having a prolonged seizure lasting more than 30 minutes should you be prepared to administer?

    A. Diazepam (Valium) 5 to 10 mg slow IV push
    B. Carbamazepine (Tegretol) 600 mg orally
    C. Phenytoin (Dilantin) 10 mg/kg IV as a loading dose
    D . Valproic acid (Depacon IV) 60 mg/kg slow IV push

Correct Answer: A.

March
2019

Monday 4	
Tuesday 5	
Wednesday 6	

Anticonvulsants

Uses:

♥ Management of epileptic seizures

♥ Treat neuropathic pain, diabetic pain, pain after shingles, fibromyalgia, migraine headaches, and bipolar disorder

March
2019

Thursday **7**	
Friday **8**	
Sat **9**	
Sun **10**	

Notes

March
2019

Monday **11**	
Tuesday **12**	
Wednesday **13**	

Anticonvulsants

Nursing Considerations:

💜 Medications should be taken around the same time each day

💜 Medications should not be stopped abruptly

💜 Anticonvulsants may increase sensitivity to sunlight and cause severe sunburn or rash

💜 Teach patient to avoid grapefruit or grapefruit juice because it may increase effect of the medication

March
2019

Thursday 14	
Friday 15	
Sat 16	
Sun 17	

Notes

March
2019

Monday **18**	
Tuesday **19**	
Wednesday **20**	

Anticonvulsants

Nursing Considerations:

♥ Medication may interfere with the effects of birth control pills – advise patients to use another form of contraceptive to avoid becoming pregnant

♥ Assess older adults taking seizure medication for abnormal heart rhythms and chest pain – report occurrences immediately

♥ Advise patients taking Klonopin to NOT smoke since this decreases the effectiveness of the medication

March
2019

Thursday 21	
Friday 22	
Sat 23	
Sun 24	

Notes

March
2019

Monday **25**	
Tuesday **26**	
Wednesday **27**	

Antidepressants – Selective Serotonin Reuptake Inhibitors (SSRIs)

Most commonly prescribed:

citalopram (Celexa)

escitalopram (Lexapro)

fluoxetine (Prozac)

paroxetine (Paxil)

sertraline (Zoloft)

March
2019

Thursday 28	
Friday 29	
Sat 30	
Sun 31	

Notes

April

Sunday	Monday	Tuesday	Wednesday
	1	2	3
7	8	9	10
14	15	16	17
21 Easter Sunday	22	23	24
28	29	30	

NCLEX Review Question

A patient who was prescribed paroxetine (Paxil) 4 weeks ago complains the medication is not working. What should the nurse respond?

A. "Increase your dose to twice a day for 2 weeks"
B. "It may take 1-8 weeks before symptoms improve"
C. "Take medicine with food for best absorption"
D. "I will speak with the provider to change medications"

Correct Answer: B.

2019

Thursday	Friday	Saturday	Notes
4	5	6	
11	12	13	
18	19 Good Friday	20	
25	26	27	

NCLEX Review Question

A parent of a child prescribed an antidepressant explains the child is experiencing unusual excitement, irritability and insomnia. The nurse expects the child is prescribed which medication?

    A. sertraline (Zoloft)
    B. duloxetine (Cymbalta)
    C. escitalopram (Lexapro)
    D . fluoxetine (Prozac)

Correct Answer: D.

April
2019

Monday 1	
Tuesday 2	
Wednesday 3	

Antidepressants – Selective Serotonin Reuptake Inhibitors (SSRIs)

Uses:

Treat moderate to major depression, obsessive-compulsive disorder (OCD), panic disorder, generalized anxiety disorder (GAD), premenstrual dysphoric disorder and post-traumatic stress disorder (PTSD)

April
2019

Thursday **4**	
Friday **5**	
Sat **6**	
Sun **7**	

Notes

April
2019

Monday **8**	
Tuesday **9**	
Wednesday **10**	

Antidepressants – Selective Serotonin Reuptake Inhibitors (SSRIs)

Nursing Considerations:

• Zoloft is the drug of choice to treat depression in elderly patients

• May take up to 4 weeks for patient to experience therapeutic effects of the medication

April
2019

Thursday 11	
Friday 12	
Sat 13	
Sun 14	

Notes

April
2019

Monday 15	

Tuesday 16	

Wednesday 17	

Antidepressants –Serotonin and Norepinephrine Reuptake Inhibitors (SNRIs)

Most commonly prescribed:

- desvenlafaxine (Pristiq)
- duloxetine (Cymbalta)
- milnacipran (Savella)
- venlafaxine (Effexor)

April
2019

Thursday 18	
Friday 19	
Sat 20	
Sun 21	

Notes

April
2019

Monday **22**	
Tuesday **23**	
Wednesday **24**	

Antidepressants –Serotonin and Norepinephrine Reuptake Inhibitors (SNRIs)

Uses:

➕ Treat major depressive disorder, panic attacks and general anxiety disorder (GAD)

➕ Cymbalta and Savella may be used to treat fibromyalgia and diabetic neuropathy

April
2019

Thursday 25	
Friday 26	
Sat 27	
Sun 28	

Notes

May

Sunday	Monday	Tuesday	Wednesday
			1
5	6	7	8
12 Mother's Day	13	14	15
19	20	21	22
26	27 Memorial Day	28	29

NCLEX Review Question

A patient who received 18 units of regular insulin an hour ago is now pale, sweaty and reports feeling anxious. What should the nurse do first?

- A. Give the patient a protein/complex carbohydrate snack.
- B. Explain this is a common side effect of insulin.
- C. Notify the prescriber immediately for an order to give IV glucose.
- D. Assess the patient's glucose level immediately.

Correct Answer: D

2019

Thursday	Friday	Saturday	Notes
2	3	4	
9	10	11	
16	17	18	
23	24	25	
30	31		

NCLEX Review Question

The nurse is preparing to administer 5 units of Novolog to a patient. What should the nurse do before administering the insulin?

    A. Look up the time the long-acting insulin was administered
    B. Assess the body area in which the last insulin dose was injected
    C. Check whether the patient's meal or snack is already on the unit
    D. Hold the dose if the patient's blood glucose level is under 110 mg/dL

Correct Answer: C

April/May
2019

Monday 29	
Tuesday 30	
Wednesday 1	

Antidepressants –Serotonin and Norepinephrine Reuptake Inhibitors (SNRIs)

Nursing Considerations:

➕ Assess patients for suicidal thoughts and behavior

➕ Monitor patient for antidepressant discontinuation syndrome which usually presents as flu-like symptoms, insomnia, and sensory disturbances

May
2019

Thursday **2**	
Friday **3**	
Sat **4**	
Sun **5**	

Notes

May
2019

Monday **6**	
Tuesday **7**	
Wednesday **8**	

Antidiabetic - Insulins

Most commonly prescribed:

☞ insulin aspart (Novolog) - rapid

☞ insulin detemir (Levemir) - long

☞ insulin glargine (Lantus) - long

☞ insulin lispro (Humalog) - rapid

May
2019

Thursday **9**	
Friday **10**	
Sat **11**	
Sun **12**	

Notes

May
2019

Monday 13	

Tuesday 14	

Wednesday 15	

Antidiabetic - Insulins

Uses:

☞ Insulin is used to treat Type 1 and 2 diabetes mellitus

Nursing Considerations:

☞ Rapid-acting insulin begins to work in about 15 minutes after injection -advise patients to eat within 5 to 10 minutes after injection

May
2019

Thursday 16	
Friday 17	
Sat 18	
Sun 19	

Notes

May
2019

Monday 20	
Tuesday 21	
Wednesday 22	

Antidiabetic - Insulins

Nursing Considerations:

☞ Regular or Short-acting insulin usually reaches the bloodstream within 30 minutes and peaks in 2 to 3 hours – Advise client to eat within 30 to 60 minutes of injection

☞ Intermediate-acting insulin generally reaches the bloodstream within 2 to 4 hours and peaks in 4 to 12 hours

May
2019

Thursday **23**	
Friday **24**	
Sat **25**	
Sun **26**	

Notes

May
2019

Monday **27**	
Tuesday **28**	
Wednesday **29**	

Antidiabetic - Insulins

Nursing Considerations:

☞ Long-acting insulin reaches the bloodstream several hours after injection and tends to lower glucose levels evenly over 24 hours – administer once daily

May/June
2019

Thursday 30	

Friday 31	

Sat 1	

Sun 2	

Notes

June

Sunday	Monday	Tuesday	Wednesday
2	3	4	5
9	10	11	12
16 Father's Day	17	18	19
23	24	25	26
30			

NCLEX Review Question

After receiving patient teaching about fexofenadine (Allegra), the patient asks the nurse if the medication should be taken during an acute asthma attack. The nurse's best response is

    A. Yes, because fexofenadine helps narrowed airways to widen and improve your effort to breathe.

    B. No, because fexofenadine causes drowsiness and may decrease your effort to breathe.

    C. Yes, because fexofenadine reduces respiratory secretions.

    D. No, because fexofenadine is used to stop hives and urticaria.

Correct Answer: B

2019

Thursday	Friday	Saturday	Notes
		1	
6	7	8	
13	14	15	
20	21	22	
27	28	29	

NCLEX Review Question

A 65-year-old male who has been prescribed diphenhydramine (Benadryl) for an allergic reaction tells the nurse he is not able to completely empty his bladder when urinating. The nurse's best response is

A. Urinary retention is a common side effect of diphenhydramine.
B. This is common medical complaint among men your age.
C. I will notify the healthcare provider for an order to stop medication.
D. I will need to perform a urinary catherization to empty your bladder

Correct Answer: C

June
2019

Monday 3	

Tuesday 4	

Wednesday 5	

Antidiabetic Oral Medications
Most commonly prescribed:

- glyburide (Diabeta, Micronase)
- metformin (Glucophage)
- pioglitazone (Actos)
- sitagliptin (Januvia)

June
2019

Thursday **6**	
Friday **7**	
Sat **8**	
Sun **9**	

Notes

June
2019

Monday **10**	
Tuesday **11**	
Wednesday **12**	

Antidiabetic Oral Medications

Uses:

Oral agents treat Type 2 diabetes mellitus

Nursing Considerations:

Oral antidiabetic medications may be used alone or in conjunction with other therapies to treat type 2 diabetes

June
2019

Thursday **13**	
Friday **14**	
Sat **15**	
Sun **16**	

Notes

June
2019

Monday 17	
Tuesday 18	
Wednesday 19	

Antidiabetic Oral Medications

Nursing Considerations:

Monitor patients taking metformin for lactic acidosis (medical emergency) which presents with symptoms such as muscle pain or weakness, numb or cold feeling in arms and legs, trouble breathing, stomach pain, nausea with vomiting, slow or uneven heart rate, dizziness, or feeling very weak or tired.

June
2019

Thursday **20**	
Friday **21**	
Sat **22**	
Sun **23**	

Notes

June
2019

Monday 24	

Tuesday 25	

Wednesday 26	

Antihistamines

Examples:

fexofenadine (Allegra)

meclizine (Antivert, Dramamine)

promethazine (Phenergan)

Uses:

Relieve allergy symptoms such as rhinitis, urticaria, and angioedema

Treat insomnia and motion sickness

June
2019

Thursday **27**	
Friday **28**	
Sat **29**	
Sun **30**	

Notes

July

Sunday	Monday	Tuesday	Wednesday
	1	2	3
7	8	9	10
14	15	16	17
21	22	23	24
28	29	30	31

NCLEX Review Question

The nurse instructs the patient who is prescribed cephalexin (Keflex) 500mg by mouth 4 times a day and an iron supplement to take the medication:

    A. 1 hour before the iron supplement
    B. 4 hours before the iron supplement
    C. 1 hour after the iron supplement
    D. With the iron supplement for better absorption.

Correct Answer: A

2019

Thursday	Friday	Saturday	Notes
4 Independence Day	5	6	
11	12	13	
18	19	20	
25	26	27	

NCLEX Review Question

The nurse is preparing to administer ciprofloxacin 400mg IV and notices the patient is also prescribed amiodarone for heart dysrhythmias. What should the nurse do before administering the medication?

    A. Ask another nurse to verify the order and then administer.
    B. Notify the healthcare provider immediately.
    C. Check to see if the patient ate their last meal
    D. Assess the patient's blood glucose level.

Correct Answer: B

July
2019

Monday 1	
Tuesday 2	
Wednesday 3	

Antihistamines

Nursing Considerations:

Advise patients to take the medication on an empty stomach with a full glass of water

Monitor elderly patients for orthostatic hypotension when taking antihistamines

July
2019

Thursday **4**	
Friday **5**	
Sat **6**	
Sun **7**	

Notes

July
2019

Monday 8	
Tuesday 9	
Wednesday 10	

Antihistamines

Nursing Considerations:

Monitor patients for symptoms of Neuroleptic Malignant Syndrome (NMS) which include a temperature greater than 106.7 degrees Fahrenheit, muscle rigidity, altered mental status, irregular pulse or blood pressure, tachycardia, diaphoresis and cardiac dysrhythmias.

July
2019

Thursday 11	
Friday 12	
Sat 13	
Sun 14	

Notes

July
2019

Monday 15	

Tuesday 16	

Wednesday 17	

Anti-infectives - Cephalosporin

Most commonly prescribed:

♥ cefdinir (Omnicef)

♥ cephalexin (Keflex)

Uses:

♥ Cephalosporins treat and prevent a wide variety of bacterial infections such as respiratory, skin, and urinary tract infections

July
2019

Thursday **18**	
Friday **19**	
Sat **20**	
Sun **21**	

Notes

July
2019

Monday 22	
Tuesday 23	
Wednesday 24	

Anti-infectives - Cephalosporin

Nursing Considerations:

Cephalosporins may be used as an alternative for clients who are allergic to penicillin

Anti-infectives - Fluoroquinolone

Most commonly prescribed:

ciprofloxacin (Cipro)

levofloxacin (Levaquin)

July
2019

Thursday **25**	
Friday **26**	
Sat **27**	
Sun **28**	

Notes

July
2019

Monday **29**	
Tuesday **30**	
Wednesday **31**	

Anti-infectives - Fluoroquinolone

Uses:

Fluoroquinolones treat a wide variety of bacterial infections such as anthrax and infections of the sinuses, skin, lungs, ears, airway, urinary tract

Nursing Considerations:

Advise patients to take medication 1 hour before meals or 2 hours after meals

August
2019

Thursday **1**	
Friday **2**	
Sat **3**	
Sun **4**	

Notes

August

Sunday	Monday	Tuesday	Wednesday
4	5	6	7
11	12	13	14
18	19	20	21
25	26	27	28

NCLEX Review Question

A patient prescribed amoxicillin (Amoxil) 250mg orally informs the nurse all the following symptoms occurred after taking the medication. Which symptom is a true allergic reaction?

    A. Upset stomach
    B. Oral thrush
    C. Foul smelling urine
    D. Hives and rash

Correct Answer: D

2019

Thursday	Friday	Saturday	Notes
1	2	3	
8	9	10	
15	16	17	
22	23	24	
29	30	31	

NCLEX Review Question

A patient who is prescribed a cephalosporin reports to the nurse a penicillin allergy. The nurse will

- A. Closely monitor the patient for an allergic reaction.
- B. Notify the healthcare provider immediately.
- C. Prepare seizure precautions
- D. Decrease the dose of the medication

Correct Answer: A

August
2019

Monday 5	
Tuesday 6	
Wednesday 7	

Anti-infectives - Macrolide

Most commonly prescribed:

azithromycin (Zithromax)

Uses:

Macrolides treat a variety of bacterial infections such as sexually transmitted infections and infections of the respiratory tract, gastrointestinal tract, and skin (severe acne). May be used to prevent endocarditis for dental procedures.

August
2019

Thursday 8	
Friday 9	
Sat 10	
Sun 11	

Notes

August
2019

Monday 12	
Tuesday 13	
Wednesday 14	

Anti-infectives - Macrolide

Nursing Considerations:

➕ Macrolides may be used as an alternative for clients who are allergic to penicillin

Anti-infectives - Penicillin

Most commonly prescribed:

- ↻ amoxicillin (Amoxil)
- ↻ penicillin (Pen-VK)

August
2019

Thursday 15	
Friday 16	
Sat 17	
Sun 18	

Notes

August
2019

Monday 19	

Tuesday 20	

Wednesday 21	

Anti-infectives - Penicillin

Uses:

↻ Penicillin treats and prevents a wide variety of bacterial infections such as streptococcal infections, syphilis and Lyme disease

Nursing Considerations:

↻ Monitor potassium levels for clients who concurrently take penicillin and potassium-sparing diuretics or ACE inhibitors because of an increased risk of hyperkalemia

August
2019

Thursday 22	
Friday 23	
Sat 24	
Sun 25	

Notes

August
2019

Monday 26	
Tuesday 27	
Wednesday 28	

Anti-infectives - Sulfonamide

Most commonly prescribed:

❧ trimethoprim-sulfamethoxazole (Septra, Bactrim)

Uses:

❧ Sulfonamides treat urinary infections, protozoal infections, and some types of bacterial pneumonia

Nursing Considerations:

❧ Advise patients taking sulfonamides that basil may affect the absorption of the medication

August
2019

Thursday **29**	
Friday **30**	
Sat **31**	
Sun **1**	

Notes

September

Sunday	Monday	Tuesday	Wednesday
1	2 Labor Day	3	4
8	9	10	11
15	16	17	18
22	23	24	25
29	30		

NCLEX Review Question

A patient who has been taking tetracycline for 5 days tells the nurse a cottage cheese-like substance has appeared on the roof of their mouth. The nurse instructs the patient to:

A. Stop taking the medication immediately.
B. Take the medication with milk or food
C. Increase water intake and avoid milk
D. Use a sterile swab to remove the substance

Correct Answer: C

2019

Thursday	Friday	Saturday	Notes
5	6	7	
12	13	14	
19	20	21	
26	27	28	

NCLEX Review Question

A patient taking aripiprazole (Abilify) 10 mg daily for 2 weeks reports to the nurse he is experiencing increased insomnia restlessness and diarrhea. What is the nurse's best response?

- A. Stop the medication immediately.
- B. Increase the dose to 15 mg daily.
- C. Keep taking the medication and symptoms should go away.
- D. Notify your healthcare provider to receive another medication.

Correct Answer: C

September
2019

Monday 2	
Tuesday 3	
Wednesday 4	

Anti-infectives - Tetracycline

Most commonly prescribed:

doxycycline (Vibramycin)

Uses:

Tetracyclines treat respiratory infections, skin infections, sexually transmitted infections (syphilis, chlamydia), urinary tract infections, gastrointestinal tract infections (Helicobacter pylori).

September
2019

Thursday 5	
Friday 6	
Sat 7	
Sun 8	

Notes

September
2019

Monday **9**	
Tuesday **10**	
Wednesday **11**	

Anti-infectives - Tetracycline

Nursing Considerations:

Tetracyclines should not be given to children under 8 years old and pregnant women due to potential of permanent staining of developing teeth and affecting the strength and shape of bones

Advise patients to take tetracyclines on an empty stomach with a full glass of water

September
2019

Thursday **12**	
Friday **13**	
Sat **14**	
Sun **15**	

Notes

September
2019

Monday 16	
Tuesday 17	
Wednesday 18	

Antipsychotics

Most commonly prescribed:

- aripiprazole (Abilify)
- olanzapine (Zyprexa)
- quetiapine (Seroquel)

September
2019

Thursday 19	
Friday 20	
Sat 21	
Sun 22	

Notes

September
2019

Monday 23	

Tuesday 24	

Wednesday 25	

Antipsychotics

Uses:

♥ Treat acute and chronic psychosis

♥ May be used to treat substance abuse, obsessive-compulsive disorder, post-traumatic disorder, depression, bipolar disorder and personality disorders

Nursing Considerations:

♥ Antipsychotic medication should never be used to chemically restrain patients who wander, have insomnia, or are uncooperative

September
2019

Thursday **26**	
Friday **27**	
Sat **28**	
Sun **29**	

Notes

September/October
2019

Monday 30	
Tuesday 1	
Wednesday 2	

Antipsychotics

Nursing Considerations:

🫀 Before giving antipsychotic medications, assess if patient is having suicidal thoughts and initiate appropriate precautions if needed

🫀 Antipsychotics can cause extrapyramidal side effects such as muscle stiffness, tremors or abnormal movements

October
2019

Thursday **3**	
Friday **4**	
Sat **5**	
Sun **6**	

Notes

October

Sunday	Monday	Tuesday	Wednesday
		1	2
6	7	8	9
13	14 Columbus Day	15	16
20	21	22	23
27	28	29	30

NCLEX Review Question

A nurse caring for a patient newly prescribed omeprazole (Prilosec) 20 mg daily is preparing patient teaching. Which of the following should the nurse include?

    A. Take medication with meals.
    B. Take medication at bedtime.
    C. Do not take daily multivitamin
    D. Take a daily multivitamin

Correct Answer: D

2019

Thursday	Friday	Saturday	Notes
3	4	5	
10	11	12	
17	18	19	
24	25	26	
31 Halloween			

NCLEX Review Question

A nurse is caring for a patient prescribed a short-acting beta agonist (SABA) as a rescue drug. Which sign or symptom indicates the patient is using the inhaler very frequently?

    A. Oral candidiasis.
    B. Tremors
    C. Urinary frequency.
    D. Dilated pupils.

Correct Answer: B

October
2019

Monday 7	

Tuesday 8	

Wednesday 9	

Antiulcer Agents

Most commonly prescribed:

amoxicillin (Amoxil)

dexlansoprazole (Dexilant)

esomeprazole (Nexium)

famotidine (Pepcid)

omeprazole (Prilosec)

pantoprazole (Protonix)

October
2019

Thursday **10**	
Friday **11**	
Sat **12**	
Sun **13**	

Notes

October
2019

Monday **14**	
Tuesday **15**	
Wednesday **16**	

Antiulcer Agents

Uses:

🔹 Treat and prevent peptic ulcer

🔹 Manage symptoms of gastroesophageal reflux disease (GERD)

🔹 A combined antibiotic and gastric acid suppression therapy may be used to treat ulcers caused by H. pylori infection

October
2019

Thursday **17**	
Friday **18**	
Sat **19**	
Sun **20**	

Notes

October
2019

Monday 21	
Tuesday 22	
Wednesday 23	

Antiulcer Agents

Nursing Considerations:

Advise patients to take gastric acid suppression agents 30 minutes to 1 hour prior to meals

Asthma Medications

Most commonly prescribed:

albuterol & ipratropium (Combivent)

albuterol (Proventil, Ventoli, Proair, Accuneb)

Montelukast (Singulair)

October
2019

Thursday 24	
Friday 25	
Sat 26	
Sun 27	

Notes

October
2019

Monday 28	

Tuesday 29	

Wednesday 30	

Asthma Medications

Uses:

Bronchodilators work by relaxing and opening the air passages to the lungs to make breathing easier – no effect on inflammation

Leukotriene receptor antagonists (LTRAs) are used to prevent wheezing, difficulty breathing, chest tightness, and coughing caused by asthma

October/November
2019

Thursday **31**	
Friday **1**	
Sat **2**	
Sun **3**	

Notes

November

Sunday	Monday	Tuesday	Wednesday
3	4	5	6
10	11 Veterans Day	12	13
17	18	19	20
24	25	26	27

NCLEX Review Question

A nursing is preparing to administer carvedilol (Coreg) 25 mg orally to a patient. Available dose is 6.25 mg/tablet. How many tablets will the nurse administer?

    A. 4 tablets
    B. 2 tablets
    C. 4.5 tablets
    D. 2.5 tablets

Correct Answer: A

2019

Thursday	Friday	Saturday	Notes
	1	2	
7	8	9	
14	15	16	
21	22	23	
28 Thanksgiving Day	29	30	

NCLEX Review Question

A nurse is caring for a patient prescribed carvedilol (Coreg) 6.25 mg twice daily? The patient reports feeling anxious and having heart palpitations. What does the nurse do first?

    A. Notify the healthcare provider immediately.
    B. Hold next dose of the medication.
    C. Obtain an EKG stat.
    D. Assess patient's blood glucose level.

Correct Answer: D

November
2019

Monday **4**	
Tuesday **5**	
Wednesday **6**	

Asthma Medications

Uses:

Short-term control treats acute attacks (bronchoconstriction related to asthma) and decrease the occurrence and intensity of future attacks which is considered long term control

November
2019

Thursday **7**	
Friday **8**	
Sat **9**	
Sun **10**	

Notes

November
2019

Monday 11	
Tuesday 12	
Wednesday 13	

Asthma Medications

Nursing Considerations:

➕ Advise patients to use Albuterol first if taking more than 1 inhalant and wait at least 5 minutes before using the next inhalant medication

➕ Advise patients that bronchodilators may cause headache, nervousness, tremors, dry mouth and increased heart rate – older adults may be more sensitive to these side effects

November
2019

Thursday 14	
Friday 15	
Sat 16	
Sun 17	

Notes

November
2019

Monday **18**	
Tuesday **19**	
Wednesday **20**	

Asthma Medications

Nursing Considerations:

➕ Check patient's breathing status after giving short-acting inhaler medications.

➕ Report severe tachycardia, a rapid rise in blood pressure or chest pain to the healthcare provider

November
2019

Thursday 21	
Friday 22	
Sat 23	
Sun 24	

Notes

November
2019

Monday **25**	
Tuesday **26**	
Wednesday **27**	

Beta Blockers

Most commonly prescribed:

- ☿ atenolol (Tenormin)

- ☿ bisoprolol (Zebeta)

- ☿ carvedilol (Coreg)

- ☿ metoprolol (Lopressor, Toprol-XL)

- ☿ nebivolol (Bystolic)

November/December
2019

Thursday 28	
Friday 29	
Sat 30	
Sun 1	

Notes

December

Sunday	Monday	Tuesday	Wednesday
1	2	3	4
8	9	10	11
15	16	17	18
22	23	24	25 Christmas
29	30	31	

NCLEX Review Question

A nurse is caring for a patient prescribed diltiazem (Cardizem) 60 mg twice daily. The patient reports symptoms of fever and achy joints. What does the nurse do first?

    A.   Notify the healthcare provider immediately.
    B.   Administer a non-steroidal anti-inflammatory drug (NSAID).
    C.   Administer acetaminophen (Tylenol).
    D.   Assess patient's blood glucose level.

Correct Answer: A

2019

Thursday	Friday	Saturday	Notes
5	6	7	
12	13	14	
19	20	21	
26	27	28	

NCLEX Review Question

A nurse is caring for a pediatric patient prescribed verapamil (Calan) 4 mg/kg/day in three divided doses. The patient weighs 54 pounds. How many mg/day will the patient receive?

    A. 32 mg/day
    B. 72 mg/day
    C. 98 mg/day
    D. 295 mg/day.

Correct Answer: C

December
2019

Monday 2	
Tuesday 3	
Wednesday 4	

Beta Blockers

Uses:

☞ Treat hypertension, congestive heart failure (CHF), left ventricle dysfunction after myocardial infarction and prophylaxis angina (not immediate relief)

☞ Treat glaucoma when given as an ophthalmic – example: timolol, (Timoptic)

☞ Prevent migraine headaches

☞ Treat situational anxiety (such as public speaking)

December
2019

Thursday **5**	
Friday **6**	
Sat **7**	
Sun **8**	

Notes

December
2019

Monday **9**	
Tuesday **10**	
Wednesday **11**	

Beta Blockers

Nursing Considerations:

☞ Monitor patient's heart rate, if less than 50 beats hold the dose and contact the healthcare provider

☞ Monitor diabetic client's blood glucose levels since the medication may mask symptoms of hypoglycemia

☞ Advise client to report any difficulty breathing immediately to the healthcare provider

December
2019

Thursday **12**	
Friday **13**	
Sat **14**	
Sun **15**	

Notes

December
2019

Monday 16	

Tuesday 17	

Wednesday 18	

Calcium Channel Blockers (CCBs)

Most commonly prescribed:

- amlodipine (Norvasc, Lotrel)

- diltiazem (Cardizem, Dilacor, Tiazac)

- verapamil (Calan, Covera, Isoptin, Verelan)

December
2019

Thursday 19	
Friday 20	
Sat 21	
Sun 22	

Notes

December
2019

Monday 23	

Tuesday 24	

Wednesday 25	

Calcium Channel Blockers (CCBs)

Uses:

◆ Treat angina, hypertension, vasospasm, atrial fibrillation (a-fib), flutter, paroxysmal supraventricular tachycardia

◆ Treat post-myocardial infarction patients who cannot tolerate beta-blockers

December
2019

Thursday **26**	
Friday **27**	
Sat **28**	
Sun **29**	

Notes

December/ January
2019/2020

Monday **30**	
Tuesday **31**	
Wednesday **1**	

Calcium Channel Blockers (CCBs)

Nursing Considerations:

❖ Patients should avoid hazardous activity until stabilized on the medication

❖ Teach patients how to assess their radial pulse and to keep a record

❖ Patients >60 years of age have increased risk of severe constipation when taking calcium channel blockers

January
2020

Thursday **2**	
Friday **3**	
Sat **4**	
Sun **5**	

Notes

January

Sunday	Monday	Tuesday	Wednesday
			1 New Year's Day
5	6	7	8
12	13	14	15
19	20 M L King Day	21	22
26	27	28	29

NCLEX Review Question

A nurse is caring for a patient who has been taking prednisone (Sterapred) 40 mg daily for the past 3 months. Which sign or symptom reported by the patient is NOT a common side effect of the medication?

    A. Thinning scalp hair.
    B. Loss of appetite.
    C. Difficulty sleeping.
    D. Fragile skin.

Correct Answer: B

2020

Thursday	Friday	Saturday	Notes
2	3	4	
9	10	11	
16	17	18	
23	24	25	
30	31		

NCLEX Review Question

A nurse is preparing teaching for a patient newly prescribed prednisolone (Orapred) 20 mg daily. What is the most important information for the nurse to include?

    A. Do not stop taking drug suddenly.
    B. The medication may mask symptoms of infection.
    C. Monitor your body temperature daily.
    D. Weigh yourself weekly to monitor fluid retention.

Correct Answer: A

January
2020

Monday **6**	
Tuesday **7**	
Wednesday **8**	

Corticosteroids

Most commonly prescribed:

- fluticasone (Flonase, Flovent)
- methylprednisolone (Medrol, Depo-Medrol)
- mometasone furoate (Nasonex)
- prednisolone (Orapred, Prelone)
- prednisone (Sterapred)

January
2020

Thursday 9	
Friday 10	
Sat 11	
Sun 12	

Notes

January
2020

Monday 13	
Tuesday 14	
Wednesday 15	

Corticosteroids

Uses:

🖊 May be taken orally or injected to treat inflammation and pain usually related to arthritis, gout, autoimmune disorders (such as lupus), and other inflammatory disorders

🖊 Given as an inhaler to treat asthma and allergies

🖊 Used topically to treat skin disorders

January
2020

Thursday **16**	
Friday **17**	
Sat **18**	
Sun **19**	

Notes

January
2020

Monday 20	
Tuesday 21	
Wednesday 22	

Corticosteroids

Nursing Considerations:

- Monitor weight and blood sugars

- Decrease sodium intake

- Eat foods high in protein, calcium, and vitamin D

- Take the medication in the morning with food – the body normally secretes cortisol in the morning

January
2020

Thursday **23**	
Friday **24**	
Sat **25**	
Sun **26**	

Notes

January
2020

Monday **27**	
Tuesday **28**	
Wednesday **29**	

Corticosteroids

Nursing Considerations:

Monitor for elevated temperature and white blood cell count (WBC) – medication suppresses inflammation as well as the immune system

January/February
2020

Thursday 30	
Friday 31	
Sat 1	
Sun 2	

Notes

February

Sunday	Monday	Tuesday	Wednesday
2	3	4	5
9	10	11	12
16	17 Presidents' Day	18	19
23	24	25	26

NCLEX Review Question

A nurse is caring for a patient prescribed furosemide (Lasix) 20 mg daily. The patient's potassium level is 3.4mEq/L. What is the best action of the nurse?

    A. Document the normal level.
    B. Administer the dose and notify the prescriber.
    C. Hold the dose and notify the prescriber.
    D. Instruct the patient to eat a banana.

Correct Answer: C

2020

Thursday	Friday	Saturday	Notes
		1	
6	7	8	
13	14 Valentine's Day	15	
20	21	22	
27	28	29	

NCLEX Review Question

A nurse is assessing a patient prescribed hydrochlorothiazide (Hydrodiuril) 50 mg daily. The patient's potassium level is 3.0 mEq/L. What is the priority assessment for the patient?

A. Temperature.
B. Blood pressure.
C. Respiratory rate.
D. Heart rate and rhythm.

Correct Answer: D

February
2020

Monday 3	
Tuesday 4	
Wednesday 5	

Diuretics

Most commonly prescribed:

♥ furosemide (Lasix)

♥ hydrochlorothiazide (Hydrodiuril)

Uses:

♥ Treat acute pulmonary edema

♥ Reduce intracranial pressure and treat hyperkalemia

♥ Treat hypertension or edema due to heart failure

February
2020

Thursday **6**	
Friday **7**	
Sat **8**	
Sun **9**	

Notes

February
2020

Monday **10**	
Tuesday **11**	
Wednesday **12**	

Diuretics

Nursing Considerations:

💓 Encourage patients to take medication early in the day since the medication increases urination

💓 Monitor blood glucose levels for diabetics since thiazide diuretics may increase blood glucose levels

February
2020

Thursday 13	
Friday 14	
Sat 15	
Sun 16	

Notes

February
2020

Monday 17	
Tuesday 18	
Wednesday 19	

Diuretics

Nursing Considerations:

🩺 Encourage patients taking a loop diuretic (ex: furosemide, Lasix) to consume foods high in potassium such as bananas and oranges

🩺 Patients taking a loop diuretic may require potassium, folic acid and vitamin B supplements

February
2020

Thursday 20	
Friday 21	
Sat 22	
Sun 23	

Notes

February
2020

Monday 24	
Tuesday 25	
Wednesday 26	

Lipid-lowering Agents
Most commonly prescribed:

- atorvastatin (Lipitor)

- colesevelam (Welchol)

- ezetimibe (Vytorin)

- pravastatin (Pravachol)

- rosuvastatin (Crestor)

- simvastatin (Zocor)

February/March
2020

Thursday 27	
Friday 28	
Sat 29	
Sun 1	

Notes

March

Sunday	Monday	Tuesday	Wednesday
1	2	3	4
8	9	10	11
15	16	17	18
22	23	24	25
29	30	31	

NCLEX Review Question

A nurse is caring for an older patient prescribed simvastatin (Zocor) 60 mg every evening. The patient reports having leg cramps. What is the nurse's best action?

    A. Administer an analgesic as ordered.
    B. Massage the patient's calf to relax the muscle.
    C. Instruct the client to limit exercise to avoid overuse of muscle.
    D. Hold next dose and notify the prescriber immediately.

Correct Answer: D

2020

Thursday	Friday	Saturday	Notes
5	6	7	
12	13	14	
19	20	21	
26	27	28	

NCLEX Review Question

A nurse is caring for a patient prescribed atorvastatin (Lipitor) 40 mg daily. Which sign/symptom reported by the patient would require immediate action by the nurse?

    A. Gray-colored stools.
    B. Flatulence.
    C. Abdominal cramps.
    D. Constipation.

Correct Answer: A

March
2020

Monday 2	
Tuesday 3	
Wednesday 4	

Lipid-lowering Agents

Uses:

Reduce blood lipids to help reduce morbidity and mortality of atherosclerotic cardiovascular disease

Reduce risk of recurrent myocardial infarction (heart attack)

March
2020

Thursday **5**	
Friday **6**	
Sat **7**	
Sun **8**	

Notes

March
2020

Monday **9**	
Tuesday **10**	
Wednesday **11**	

Lipid-lowering Agents
Nursing Considerations:

• Liver function tests recommended every 12 weeks

• After a patient begins taking a statin drug, be sure to monitor for signs of rhabdomyolysis: muscle pain in the shoulders, thighs, or lower back; muscle weakness or trouble moving arms and legs; and dark red or brown urine or decreased urination

• "Statin" drugs are usually more effective when taken in the evening

March
2020

Thursday **12**	
Friday **13**	
Sat **14**	
Sun **15**	

Notes

March
2020

Monday 16	
Tuesday 17	
Wednesday 18	

Non-Steroidal Anti-Inflammatory Drugs (NSAIDS)

Most commonly prescribed:

celecoxib (Celebrex)

ibuprofen (Motrin, Advil)

naproxen (Aleve, Naprosyn)

Uses:

Management of mild to moderate pain, reduce fever, treat inflammatory disorders such as osteoarthritis, and primary dysmenorrhea

March
2020

Thursday 19	
Friday 20	
Sat 21	
Sun 22	

Notes

March
2020

Monday 23	
Tuesday 24	
Wednesday 25	

Non-Steroidal Anti-Inflammatory Drugs (NSAIDS)
Nursing Considerations:

➕ Advise patients to avoid taking with aspirin and alcohol – may cause GI bleeding

➕ Take medication with 8 oz. glass of water or with food/milk if patient experiences an upset stomach

➕ Due to increased risk of bleeding while taking NSAID, advise patients to stop medication 1 week prior to surgery

March
2020

Thursday 26	
Friday 27	
Sat 28	
Sun 29	

Notes

March/April
2020

Monday 30	

Tuesday 31	

Wednesday 1	

Sedatives/Hypnotics

Most commonly prescribed:

- diazepam (Valium)
- eszopiclone (Lunesta)
- hydroxyzine (Atarax, Vistaril)
- lorazepam (Ativan)
- promethazine (Phenergan)
- zolpidem (Ambien)

April
2020

Thursday 2	
Friday 3	
Sat 4	
Sun 5	

Notes

April

Sunday	Monday	Tuesday	Wednesday
			1
5	6	7	8
12 Easter Sunday	13	14	15
19	20	21	22
26	27	28	29

NCLEX Review Question

A nurse is discharging to home a patient who had a hip replacement and is prescribed celecoxib (Celebrex) 400 mg daily x 7 days. What precaution is most important to teach patient?

- A. Do not increase dose of this drug.
- B. Do not shave while taking this drug.
- C. Do not consume caffeine while taking this drug.
- D. Do not stop taking the drug immediately.

Correct Answer: A

2020

Thursday	Friday	Saturday	Notes
2	3	4	
9	10 Good Friday	11	
16	17	18	
23	24	25	
30			

NCLEX Review Question

A nurse is caring for a patient who recently had oral surgery and is prescribed ibuprofen (Advil) 800 mg twice daily x 7 days. Which response by the patient confirms the medication is effective?

    A. I can tolerate eating soft foods.
    B. I cannot believe the puffiness of my cheeks.
    C. My forehead feels warm
    D. My surgical incision is red.

Correct Answer: A

April
2020

Monday **6**	
Tuesday **7**	
Wednesday **8**	

Sedatives/Hypnotics

Uses:

❖ Short term relief of insomnia

❖ Sedation prior to procedures

❖ May also be used to treat seizures, skeletal muscle pain from injury, and as an adjunct for alcohol withdrawal syndrome

❖ Vistaril relieves itching due to allergies, chronic urticaria, histamine-mediated itch or dermatitis (eczema).

April
2020

Thursday 9	
Friday 10	
Sat 11	
Sun 12	

Notes

April
2020

Monday **13**	
Tuesday **14**	
Wednesday **15**	

Sedatives/Hypnotics

Nursing Considerations:

🔖 Drowsiness, unsteadiness on standing, "drugged" feeling, lightheadedness, and headache, are the most commonly reported side effects.

🔖 Grapefruit juice or grapefruit products may increase blood levels of Valium; avoid concurrent use.

🔖 Some patients using Lunesta or Ambien have reported having no memory of engaging in activities such as driving, eating, or making phone calls.

April
2020

Thursday 16	
Friday 17	
Sat 18	
Sun 19	

Notes

April
2020

Monday **20**	
Tuesday **21**	
Wednesday **22**	

Skeletal Muscle Relaxants

Most commonly prescribed:

- carisoprodol (Soma, Soprodal, Vanadom)
- cyclobenzaprine (Flexaril)
- diazepam (Valium)

April
2020

Thursday 23	
Friday 24	
Sat 25	
Sun 26	

Notes

April
2020

Monday 27	
Tuesday 28	
Wednesday 29	

Skeletal Muscle Relaxants

Uses:

🖊 An adjunct to rest and physical therapy for relief of muscle spasm associated with acute, painful musculoskeletal conditions

🖊 Treat spasticity with spinal cord diseases such as cerebral palsy or multiple sclerosis

April/May
2020

Thursday **30**	
Friday **1**	
Sat **2**	
Sun **3**	

Notes

May
2020

Monday 4	
Tuesday 5	
Wednesday 6	

Skeletal Muscle Relaxants

Nursing Considerations:

Flexaril should only be used short-term (for periods of up to two to three weeks).

May
2020

Thursday 7	
Friday 8	
Sat 9	
Sun 10	

Notes

May

Sunday	Monday	Tuesday	Wednesday
3	4	5	6
10 Mother's Day	11	12	13
17	18	19	20
24	25 Memorial Day	26	27
31			

NCLEX Review Question

A nurse is caring for a patient prescribed cyclobenzaprine (Flexaril) 10 mg three times daily? The patient reports experiencing increased dry mouth. What is the best action of the nurse?

    A. Notify the prescriber the patient is having an anticholinergic response to the medication.
    B. Obtain a urine specimen to determine hydration status.
    C. Assess the patient for orthostatic hypotension.
    D. Inform the patient this is an expected side effect of the medication.

Correct Answer: D

2020

Thursday	Friday	Saturday	Notes
	1	2	
7	8	9	
14	15	16	
21	22	23	
28	29	30	

NCLEX Review Question

A nurse is caring for a patient prescribed cyclobenzaprine (Flexaril) 10 mg three times daily. Upon reviewing the patient's medical history, which diagnosis would most concern the nurse?

    A. History of substance abuse.
    B. History of seizures.
    C. Sulfa allergy.
    D. Hypotension.

Correct Answer: B

May
2020

Monday **11**	
Tuesday **12**	
Wednesday **13**	

Skeletal Muscle Relaxants
Nursing Considerations:

✎ Interaction with other drugs that also increase serotonin (such as antidepressants, tramadol, and St. John's Wort) may cause serotonin syndrome. Symptoms of serotonin syndrome include mental status changes (such as agitation, hallucinations, coma, delirium), fast heart rate, dizziness, flushing, muscle tremor or rigidity and stomach symptoms (including nausea, vomiting, and diarrhea).

May
2020

Thursday 14	
Friday 15	
Sat 16	
Sun 17	

Notes

May
2020

Monday 18	

Tuesday 19	

Wednesday 20	

May
2020

Thursday **21**	
Friday **22**	
Sat **23**	
Sun **24**	

Notes

May
2020

Monday **25**	
Tuesday **26**	
Wednesday **27**	

NCLEX Coaching Services

Prepare to take the NCLEX in 6 weeks or less with our NCLEX Coaching package. You will have access to nursing content, question bank, daily motivation calls and weekly 1:1 coaching calls.

This service is ideal for first-time test takers with test anxiety and for those who were not successful in a previous NCLEX testing experience.

andreasnotes.com

May
2020

Thursday 28	
Friday 29	
Sat 30	
Sun 31	

Notes

Andrea's Notes is a group coaching service that offers a variety of resources to help you successfully complete nursing school and prepare for NCLEX.

We provide access to weekly live reviews, video library, nursing cheat sheets, weekly live question and answer sessions and so much more!

andreasnotes.com

Ready to cut your study time in half?

Checkout more study notes and

courses at

andreasnotes.com

We give you the support you need to

reach your nursing education and

career goals!

Made in the USA
San Bernardino, CA
27 January 2019